CORE WORKOUTS FOR SENIORS

Building Strength, Balance, and Vitality at Any Age

Basil U

COPYRIGHT

TABLE OF CONTENTS

ABOUT THE BOOK

Aging doesn't mean losing strength or giving up on fitness goals. In fact, maintaining core strength is crucial to aging gracefully and independently. Core Workouts for Seniors: Ageless Abs* is a comprehensive guide specifically designed to empower older adults to take control of their physical well-being by building a strong core. This book provides a step-by-step roadmap for achieving better balance, improved posture, reduced back pain, and enhanced mobility—all through carefully crafted core exercises that are safe, effective, and accessible to seniors of all fitness levels.

Why Core Strength Matters as We Age

Your core is the powerhouse of your body. It's made up of several important muscles, including the abdominals, obliques, lower back, and hips, all working together to support your spine, maintain stability, and power your movements. As we age, these muscles can weaken, leading to a host of issues, from poor posture and balance problems to increased risk of falls and chronic back pain. This book dives deep into why maintaining core strength becomes even more vital in later years and how doing so can dramatically improve your quality of life.

Myths Debunked: Core Workouts Are for All Ages

One of the biggest misconceptions about fitness is that core exercises are too strenuous for older adults. This couldn't be further from the truth. *Core Workouts for Seniors: Ageless Abs* breaks down these myths and offers clear, actionable insights into how seniors can safely engage in core training. Each workout is designed with modifications and adaptations, ensuring that even those with mobility issues, arthritis, or joint pain can participate.

A Tailored Approach: Beginner to Advanced Core Workouts

Whether you're new to exercising or have been active for years, this book offers core workouts that are carefully graded to suit your fitness level. Beginning with gentle movements like seated marches and pelvic tilts, progressing through intermediate exercises such as bird-dogs and knee lifts, and advancing to more challenging routines like stability ball crunches and side planks, there's something for everyone. What sets this book apart is the personalized approach it takes, providing modifications for different physical needs and abilities, ensuring that everyone—no matter where they are starting from—can benefit from the routines.

Holistic Health: Flexibility, Balance, and Endurance

Core strength alone is not enough for overall wellness. This book teaches the importance of balancing core exercises with flexibility and endurance training. You'll find guidance on how to combine these elements into a well-rounded routine that supports all aspects of senior fitness. With customizable weekly workout plans, readers can build a fitness routine that fits seamlessly into their lifestyle, with options for varied difficulty levels and specific goals such as improving balance or reducing back pain.

Overcoming Mental and Physical Barriers

Starting a new fitness routine can feel overwhelming, especially as we get older. Concerns like fear of injury, low energy, or simply feeling too old to start are common. *Core Workouts for Seniors: Ageless Abs* addresses these mental hurdles head-on, offering encouragement and practical strategies to help you overcome them. The book emphasizes building confidence through consistency, realistic goal-setting, and celebrating the small victories along the way. You'll find advice on how to incorporate core-strengthening exercises into daily life, whether it's during activities like standing up from a chair, walking, or even while watching TV.

Fueling Your Body: Nutrition and Recovery

Exercise is only part of the equation. This book highlights the critical role that nutrition and hydration play in maintaining muscle health and core strength. Seniors will learn how to fuel their bodies with a balanced diet rich in protein, healthy fats, and essential vitamins, along with practical tips for staying hydrated. Recovery is just as important as the workout itself, and the book provides valuable insights into how proper rest, stretching, and hydration help prevent injury and enhance performance. For those interested in mind-body practices, there's also a dedicated section on yoga and Pilates, offering low-impact ways to improve core strength, flexibility, and mindfulness.

Staying Motivated: Long-Term Fitness Success

One of the key challenges in any fitness journey is staying motivated over time. *Core Workouts for Seniors: Ageless Abs* doesn't just stop at teaching exercises—it offers tools and tips for maintaining long-term commitment. From mixing up your routines to keeping things fun with a workout buddy, this book helps you stay engaged in your fitness goals. With an emphasis on setting new goals as you progress, you'll find ways to keep your core workout exciting and aligned with your evolving fitness level.

Real-Life Success Stories

Nothing is more inspiring than hearing from real people who have been through the journey. In this book, you'll find stories of seniors who have transformed their lives through core training. These success stories, filled with personal anecdotes and testimonials, offer motivation and proof that it's never too late to start working on your core strength. They also provide real-life examples of how building a strong core can enhance mobility, improve posture, and increase overall confidence.

Safety First: Injury Prevention and Expert Guidance

Safety is a top priority in any exercise routine, especially for seniors. The book teaches readers how to avoid injury by using proper form, recognizing the signs of overtraining, and listening to their bodies. Detailed diagrams and descriptions ensure that readers can follow along with exercises safely. And for those with specific concerns or pre-existing conditions, the book offers advice on when it might be necessary to consult a physical therapist or a fitness professional for guidance.

Your Journey to Ageless Abs Starts Here

Ultimately, *Core Workouts for Seniors: Ageless Abs* is more than just an exercise guide—it's a holistic approach to senior fitness that empowers you to build and maintain core strength at any age. By following the advice and workouts laid out in this book, you will gain more than just physical benefits. You will improve your mental well-being, increase your confidence, and enjoy a greater sense of independence as you age.

This book is an invitation to take ownership of your health, to challenge misconceptions about aging, and to discover what your body is truly capable of, no matter how many birthdays you've celebrated. Whether you're looking to reduce back pain, prevent falls, improve your balance, or simply feel stronger, this book is your trusted companion on the path to lifelong fitness. Your journey to achieving ageless abs begins now!

INTRODUCTION

Aging brings many physical changes, but one that often goes unnoticed is the gradual weakening of our core muscles. Our core—the group of muscles that include our abdominals, lower back, and pelvic muscles—plays an essential role in nearly every movement we make. Whether it's standing up from a chair, bending over to tie a shoe, or simply maintaining good posture, these muscles are at work every day, supporting and stabilizing the body.

For seniors, core strength becomes even more critical. A strong core enhances balance, making us less prone to falls, which are a leading cause of injury in older adults. With improved stability, you can enjoy greater freedom in your movements—whether that means taking a brisk walk in the park or comfortably playing with your grandkids on the floor. Beyond mobility, a strong core can also reduce common aches and pains, particularly in the lower back. The connection between core strength and overall health is undeniable, and maintaining or improving this area of your body as you age is one of the best investments you can make for a vibrant, independent life.

But it's not just about physical health. Strengthening your core is also linked to mental well-being. There's something profoundly empowering about regaining control over your body's movements, especially when society often suggests that we should expect to slow down as we age. Instead of giving in to the decline, strengthening your core can help you maintain the active, fulfilling life you deserve.

Debunking Myths: Core Exercises Are for All Ages

One of the biggest misconceptions surrounding fitness for seniors is the belief that core workouts are too strenuous or advanced for older adults. Perhaps you've seen intense fitness programs with seemingly impossible ab exercises and thought, "I could never do that." Or maybe you've been told that it's too late to start, that once we hit a certain age, the decline in strength and muscle mass is inevitable.

Let me reassure you—core exercises are not just for the young or elite athletes. In fact, they are for everyone, especially seniors. The truth is that core workouts can be tailored to fit any age or ability level. You don't need to do hundreds of crunches or perform complex routines that leave you sore for days. Instead, gentle yet effective exercises can be incorporated into your daily life, helping you rebuild strength without the risk of injury.

This book is here to challenge the myth that core exercises are out of reach for older adults. You can work on your abs and overall core, regardless of your starting point. From simple seated exercises that can be done in a chair to more advanced moves that you can progress to over time, this book offers a range of options for every senior looking to improve their core strength.

The message is clear: core exercises are for all ages. If you've been holding back from working on your core because you believe it's too late, think again. This book will show you how to build a strong, stable core in a way that fits your unique needs, abilities, and lifestyle.

How This Book Will Help You Achieve Ageless Abs

So, what exactly can you expect from this book? *Core Workouts for Seniors: Ageless Abs* is designed to guide you through a safe, effective, and empowering journey to strengthen your core and improve your quality of life. Whether you're a fitness beginner or someone with some experience, this book will help you achieve core strength in a way that feels manageable and, most importantly, sustainable.

First, we'll start by exploring the core muscles and why they matter—beyond just aesthetics. You'll learn how your core supports everyday movements, from walking to standing up straight, and how improving this area can have far-reaching benefits for your overall health. We'll also address common questions and concerns, such as how often you should work out your core, how to modify exercises if you have back or joint issues, and what kind of results you can expect to see over time.

Next, we'll dive into the workouts themselves. This book offers exercises suited for all fitness levels. For those just starting out, we'll begin with beginner-friendly moves that are gentle on your joints and back. Chair-based exercises will be introduced for those who prefer seated routines, making them accessible even if you have mobility concerns. As you progress, we'll build up to more challenging exercises, ensuring that you continue to make gains in strength and endurance.

Along the way, you'll hear from real people who have transformed their bodies and lives through core training. Their stories will show you what's possible when you commit to building a stronger core, and how these workouts can lead to greater independence, confidence, and physical freedom.

Finally, we'll discuss how to incorporate these workouts into your daily routine, making them a seamless part of your life. Core exercises don't have to take hours out of your day. With the right mindset and commitment, you can work these movements into simple activities—whether it's standing at the kitchen counter or taking a walk around your neighborhood.

This book isn't about sculpting a six-pack. It's about building strength, stability, and resilience. You'll be empowered to take control of your physical health at any age and develop a strong core that supports you through all of life's activities. By the end of this journey, you'll not only feel the physical benefits of core workouts, but you'll also experience a renewed sense of vitality, confidence, and independence.

What's Next?

As you turn the page, we'll start by diving into the fundamentals: understanding the core muscles and why they are so important to your overall well-being. From there, we'll guide you step-by-step through the exercises, providing clear instructions, modifications, and tips to ensure you're comfortable and confident in every move. The goal is to empower you with knowledge and tools to make core workouts a regular part of your routine, allowing you to reap the long-term benefits of a strong, resilient core.

Ageless abs may sound like a lofty goal, but with the right mindset and dedication, it's entirely within your reach. This book will be your companion on the journey to stronger, healthier abs, no matter where you're starting from. Let's begin this exciting chapter of your fitness journey together!

CHAPTER 1

UNDERSTANDING YOUR CORE: MORE THAN JUST ABS

When most people think of the core, their minds immediately jump to the abdominal muscles—the ones that form the six-pack we often associate with fitness. But the truth is, the core is much more than just abs. It's an intricate system of muscles that work together to support and stabilize your body, allowing you to move efficiently and protect your spine. For seniors, maintaining strength in this crucial area is essential for mobility, balance, and overall quality of life.

What Exactly Is the Core?

The core is like the foundation of a house—it holds everything together. While the abdominal muscles certainly play a role, they're only one piece of the puzzle. The core consists of a complex network of muscles, each contributing to the stability and movement of your entire body.

- Rectus Abdominis: These are the famous "six-pack" muscles that run down the front of your abdomen. They're responsible for flexing your spine, such as when you bend forward.
- Obliques: Located on the sides of your abdomen, the obliques come in two types: internal and external. They help you twist and bend from side to side, and they're essential for stabilizing the trunk during various movements.

- Transverse Abdominis: Often referred to as the body's natural corset, the transverse abdominis lies deep beneath the other abdominal muscles and wraps around the spine for protection. This muscle is vital for maintaining stability and balance.

- Lower Back Muscles (Erector Spinae): These muscles run along the spine and are key players in keeping your posture upright. They help you stand tall, sit up straight, and provide support during lifting and other movements.

- Hip Muscles: The hips, including muscles like the hip flexors and glutes, are often overlooked when people think of the core. However, they play a crucial role in movement, stability, and alignment. Strong hip muscles can also help prevent falls by keeping you steady on your feet.

All these muscles work together to support your body's movements. Whether you're walking, bending, or even sitting, your core is constantly engaged to help you stay balanced and stable.

Why Core Strength Matters for Seniors

As we age, maintaining core strength becomes increasingly important for a number of reasons. First and foremost, a strong core helps improve "posture". Many seniors experience a forward-hunched posture due to years of weak core muscles, leading to back pain and a less confident stance. By strengthening your core, you can stand taller, walk with more ease, and alleviate some of the pressure that may accumulate in your spine and lower back.

A strong core also significantly reduces "back pain"—a common complaint among older adults. Weak core muscles force the lower back to take on too much responsibility, leading to strain and discomfort. When the core is strong, it helps distribute the workload more evenly, reducing the risk of injury and discomfort.

Beyond posture and back health, core strength plays a crucial role in "balance and stability" . For seniors, maintaining good balance is essential to prevent falls. Falls are one of the leading causes of injury in older adults, often resulting in fractures or more serious health problems. The core muscles help to stabilize your body, allowing you to recover more quickly if you trip or lose your footing. When your core is strong, you're better equipped to move confidently and react swiftly to maintain your balance, no matter the situation.

Take, for instance, the story of "Betty", a 72-year-old who had struggled with balance for years. She would often avoid activities that required her to walk on uneven surfaces, out of fear of falling. After working on her core strength for a few months, Betty noticed a dramatic improvement—not only in her balance but in her confidence. She began enjoying outdoor walks again and even joined a local hiking group, something she never thought she'd do in her 70s. This transformation didn't require hours of strenuous exercise; it was simply the result of consistent core-focused movements tailored to her abilities.

For those dealing with chronic conditions like "osteoporosis" or "arthritis ", core strength can also provide relief. These conditions often affect posture and movement, making it difficult to maintain an active lifestyle. Strengthening the core muscles can help alleviate pressure on the spine and joints, leading to improved flexibility and a wider range of motion. When you strengthen the muscles that support your body, you're giving your bones and joints the backup they need to carry you through the day.

Common Challenges Seniors Face in Maintaining Core Strength

While the benefits of core strength are clear, maintaining it can become challenging with age. One of the most significant barriers is "muscle loss". As we grow older, we naturally lose muscle mass—a condition known as sarcopenia. This loss is often gradual and subtle but becomes more pronounced as we enter our senior years. With less muscle mass, it becomes harder to perform activities that once seemed effortless, like standing up from a chair or reaching for something on a high shelf.

In addition to muscle loss, many seniors experience decreased flexibility. Tight or stiff muscles, particularly in the hips and lower back, can limit mobility and make certain core exercises feel uncomfortable. This can discourage many older adults from engaging in activities that require stretching or bending. But here's the good news: flexibility can be improved, even in your golden years. Gentle core exercises that focus on stretching, combined with mindful movements, can help you regain some of the flexibility you may have lost.

Another common challenge is fear of injury. Understandably, many seniors are cautious about starting a new exercise routine, especially if they've dealt with injuries in the past. Concerns about straining the back or aggravating an existing condition often prevent older adults from working on their core. However, core workouts don't have to be risky. In fact, when done correctly, they can help prevent injury by improving muscle support and reducing the risk of falls.

For instance, consider Tom, a 68-year-old who had undergone surgery for a herniated disc years earlier. After his surgery, he became hesitant to exercise, fearing that he might re-injure his back. Eventually, he started a simple core-strengthening routine, beginning with chair exercises that didn't put too much strain on his spine. Over time, Tom not only strengthened his core but also experienced less pain and increased mobility, allowing him to return to activities he loved, like gardening and playing with his grandchildren.

The key to overcoming these challenges is consistency. It's important to start slowly and choose exercises that are appropriate for your current level of fitness. Even if you've been inactive for years, it's never too late to begin working on your core. By addressing muscle loss and improving flexibility through targeted exercises, you'll not only strengthen your core but also regain confidence in your ability to move freely.

By understanding the components of your core and the benefits that come with strengthening these muscles, you're taking the first step toward better balance, posture, and mobility. In the next chapter, we'll delve into specific exercises that are safe, effective, and tailored to seniors. Whether you're just starting your fitness journey or looking to improve your current routine, you'll find a wide range of options to suit your needs. Let's get ready to transform your core—and your life.

CHAPTER 2

GETTING STARTED: CORE WORKOUT BASICS FOR SENIORS

Before diving into any workout routine, it's essential to have a clear understanding of where you're starting from and what your body needs. Whether you've been active for years or are just now returning to exercise, this chapter will guide you through assessing your current fitness level, offer important safety precautions, and help you determine if you need any equipment for your core workouts. Remember, building a strong core is a journey, and this is where it all begins.

Assessing Your Fitness Level

Knowing your fitness level helps ensure that you start at a pace that's right for you, reducing the risk of injury and frustration. There's no need for complicated tests—simple self-assessments can provide all the information you need to get started.

1. Chair Sit-and-Stand Test

This test is a great way to assess the strength of your lower body and core, both of which are essential for balance and stability. Here's how to do it:

- Sit on a sturdy chair with your feet flat on the ground and arms crossed over your chest.

- Try to stand up from the chair without using your hands.

- Sit back down and repeat the motion as many times as you can in 30 seconds.

If you can complete 8-12 repetitions, that's a good indicator that your lower body and core are in fair shape. If you struggle to stand up without using your hands, don't worry—this just means you'll want to start with gentler exercises.

2. Plank Test (Modified Version)

The plank is one of the best exercises for testing core strength. A full plank may be too challenging initially, but a modified version will still give you a sense of where your core strength stands.

- Start by positioning yourself on your hands and knees, then lower your forearms to the ground so that you're in a modified plank position, keeping your back straight.
- Hold this position for as long as you can, aiming for at least 15-20 seconds.

If you find it difficult to maintain good form for more than a few seconds, that's completely normal. Many seniors may struggle with core endurance at first. The goal is simply to see where you're starting, and over time, you'll improve.

3. Balance Test

Balance is a key indicator of core strength, and this simple test will give you a sense of your current abilities:

- Stand near a sturdy surface like a counter or chair in case you need support.

- Lift one foot off the ground and see how long you can balance on one leg. Try to hold this position for at least 10 seconds without wobbling or needing to grab onto the support.

If you find it hard to balance for more than a few seconds, it's a sign that your core and stabilizing muscles could use some attention. Don't be discouraged—core workouts can greatly improve your balance with consistent practice.

These simple assessments will help you understand your starting point and give you a clearer picture of where to focus your efforts. It's important to remember that there's no "right" or "wrong" result here—just an honest assessment of where you are today so you can build from there.

Key Precautions and Modifications for Senior Core Workouts

One of the most important things to keep in mind when starting a core workout routine is safety. Your body has been through decades of wear and tear, and it's important to respect that. Taking precautions and modifying exercises to suit your fitness level will ensure that you build strength safely and avoid injury.

1. Protect Your Joints

For many seniors, joint pain—especially in the knees, hips, and lower back—can be a barrier to exercise. The good news is that core workouts can be done in ways that are gentle on the joints. Here are a few tips:

- Use a chair for support: If standing exercises feel unstable or uncomfortable, try doing modified versions seated in a chair. Chair-based exercises can still activate your core while reducing pressure on your knees and back.

- Avoid high-impact movements: There's no need to jump or perform fast, jerky motions. Slow, controlled movements are just as effective and far easier on your joints.

- Incorporate stretching: Stretching both before and after your workout will keep your muscles and joints flexible, reducing the risk of strain or stiffness.

2. Focus on Form

Proper form is crucial when it comes to core exercises, especially for seniors. Performing movements with incorrect form can lead to injury or strain, particularly in the lower back.

- Engage your core: Whether you're sitting, standing, or lying down, always focus on keeping your core muscles engaged. Imagine pulling your belly button toward your spine—this will help you activate the right muscles.

- Don't rush: There's no need to power through your exercises. In fact, slow and steady wins the race when it comes to core workouts. Performing each movement slowly ensures that you're using the right muscles and maintaining good form.

- Take breaks: Listen to your body. If an exercise feels too challenging or if you're feeling fatigued, take a break. It's better to rest and come back to the exercise with good form than to push through and risk injury.

3. Modify to Your Fitness Level

Every exercise can be adapted to suit your current abilities. For example, if you find it difficult to hold a plank, start with a modified version on your knees rather than your toes. If standing exercises are tough on your balance, try holding onto the back of a chair for support. The goal is to gradually increase your strength and endurance, not to jump into advanced moves right away.

Let's look at Ron's story for some inspiration. At 70, Ron had struggled with lower back pain for years and was hesitant to try core exercises. He started with modified versions of each exercise, doing them slowly and with the support of a chair. Over time, his core grew stronger, his back pain decreased, and he gained more confidence in his movements. Today, he's able to do full planks and enjoys a wide range of physical activities without fear of injury.

Choosing the Right Equipment: Do You Need It?

One of the first questions many seniors ask when starting a core workout routine is, "Do I need special equipment?" The answer depends on your preferences and fitness level, but the good news is that you can achieve excellent results with little to no equipment.

1. Bodyweight Exercises

For many seniors, bodyweight exercises are more than enough to build core strength. Movements like planks, bridges, and seated twists rely on your body's own weight to provide resistance. These exercises are great because they can be done anywhere—no gym or fancy equipment required.

2. Resistance Bands

If you're looking to add a bit more challenge to your workouts, resistance bands are a fantastic option. They're inexpensive, easy to store, and provide varying levels of resistance to suit your needs. Resistance bands can be used to add intensity to exercises like seated twists or leg lifts, helping you build strength without putting strain on your joints.

3. Stability Balls

Stability balls (also known as exercise balls) can be useful for core workouts, as they force your muscles to engage in order to maintain balance. However, if you're just starting out or have balance issues, you may want to hold off on using a stability ball until you feel more confident in your abilities. Stability balls are best suited for more advanced exercises, so consider them an option down the road.

4. Small Weights

For those looking to incorporate more resistance, small hand weights (1-3 pounds) can be a great addition. You can use them during seated or standing exercises to add a little extra challenge. However, like the stability ball, weights aren't necessary for beginners. Bodyweight exercises alone can provide all the resistance you need when starting out.

In short, you don't need a gym full of equipment to strengthen your core. Whether you choose to keep it simple with bodyweight exercises or add in a few tools like resistance bands or small weights, the key is finding what works for you. As you progress, you can experiment with different pieces of equipment to keep your workouts engaging and challenging.

CHAPTER 3

THE BENEFITS OF CORE WORKOUTS FOR SENIORS

As we age, maintaining physical strength isn't just about looking good—it's about staying independent, preventing injuries, and enjoying daily life with ease. Core workouts are especially important for seniors because they offer benefits that go far beyond aesthetics. In this chapter, we'll explore how a strong core can improve balance and stability, enhance posture and reduce back pain, and even boost confidence and independence. Each benefit contributes to a more active, fulfilling life.

Improved Balance and Stability

One of the most common concerns as we grow older is the risk of falling. Falls can lead to serious injuries, and many seniors worry about how a fall might impact their independence. The good news is that a strong core can be your greatest ally in preventing falls.

How Core Exercises Prevent Falls

The muscles in your core—especially the deep stabilizing muscles in your abdomen, hips, and lower back—play a critical role in balance. They act like a support system for your entire body, helping you stay steady on your feet. When these muscles are weak, it's much easier to lose your balance, especially when doing activities that require coordination or moving quickly, like walking upstairs or bending over to pick something up.

By regularly performing core exercises, you train your body to react more quickly and maintain stability. This is essential for seniors because everyday activities, such as getting out of bed, reaching for something on a shelf, or even walking on uneven ground, require balance and coordination. A strong core gives you the control needed to keep your body upright, reducing the chances of falls.

Real-Life Impact: Helen's Story

Take **Helen**, for example. At 68, she was active but found herself becoming increasingly unsteady. Simple tasks like walking on wet pavement or standing up from a chair felt risky. After a few months of doing gentle core exercises, Helen noticed a significant improvement. She could move more confidently, her balance was better, and her fear of falling lessened. Her newfound stability allowed her to walk her dog in the park without constantly worrying about tripping or falling.

Helen's story is just one example of how strengthening your core can transform the way you move through life, making everyday activities safer and more manageable.

Enhanced Posture and Reduced Back Pain

Another major benefit of core workouts is improved posture. Good posture isn't just about standing tall—it's about aligning your body so that your muscles and joints work together efficiently, without straining any particular area. Unfortunately, many seniors experience a gradual decline in posture as they age, leading to slouching, rounded shoulders, and a forward-leaning stance. This decline in posture often results in back pain, particularly in the lower back.

How Core Strength Supports Posture

Your core muscles, especially those in the abdomen and lower back, provide support for your spine. When these muscles are weak, the spine doesn't have the support it needs, leading to poor posture and an increased risk of back pain. Strengthening the core helps to realign the spine, reducing pressure on the vertebrae and improving posture.

Better posture doesn't just make you look more youthful and confident; it also eases strain on your muscles and joints. With a strong core, you'll find that sitting, standing, and even walking for long periods become much more comfortable.

How Core Exercises Reduce Back Pain

Back pain is a common issue for seniors, but it doesn't have to be a permanent part of aging. In fact, many people experience relief from chronic back pain simply by strengthening their core. The muscles in your lower back, when properly trained, can provide the support needed to take pressure off your spine.

For example, exercises like pelvic tilts and bridges work the muscles in your lower back and abdomen simultaneously, helping to relieve tension in the back. Over time, these exercises can not only reduce pain but also prevent future flare-ups by building a protective "corset" of strength around your spine.

Real-Life Impact: Tom's Story

Tom, a 72-year-old retiree, had dealt with lower back pain for years. He'd tried different therapies and medications, but nothing seemed to provide lasting relief. His doctor suggested that his weak core might be contributing to the problem. Hesitant at first, Tom started incorporating gentle core exercises into his routine. Within a few weeks, he noticed a significant reduction in his pain. By focusing on strengthening his core muscles, Tom was able to take pressure off his spine, improve his posture, and enjoy a pain-free life.

Boosting Confidence and Independence

The physical benefits of core workouts are obvious, but what often gets overlooked is how these exercises can also improve your mental and emotional well-being. A strong core can lead to greater self-reliance, enhanced confidence, and a more positive body image—especially for seniors who may feel like their bodies aren't as capable as they once were.

How Core Strength Enhances Self-Reliance

One of the greatest gifts core workouts offers is the ability to take control of your physical health. As we age, many people fear losing their independence, whether it's needing help with daily tasks or relying on others for mobility. Strengthening your core can help you maintain independence longer, allowing you to perform daily activities without assistance.

Imagine being able to get up from a chair, carry groceries, or climb stairs with ease. These are things that many take for granted, but as we age, they can become more difficult. A strong core gives you the strength and stability to tackle these tasks on your own, helping you feel more self-reliant and capable.

Boosting Confidence Through Fitness

There's something incredibly empowering about feeling strong, regardless of your age. Core workouts can help you regain a sense of control over your body, boosting your confidence in your physical abilities. This is especially true for seniors who may have spent years dealing with injuries, illness, or the natural effects of aging.

When you feel strong in your core, you're more likely to stand taller, move with purpose, and approach life's challenges with confidence. This increased sense of self-assurance doesn't just impact your physical health—it has a ripple effect on your emotional well-being, improving your overall outlook on life.

Positive Body Image at Any Age

It's never too late to appreciate and celebrate what your body can do. Core workouts not only help you feel stronger, but they also encourage a positive body image. As you progress through your core exercises, you may notice changes in how your body feels and functions. Even small improvements can lead to a greater sense of satisfaction and pride in your physical abilities.

Real-Life Impact: Maria's Story

Maria, at 74, never thought she'd feel confident about her body again. After years of neglecting her physical health, she didn't feel strong or capable. But after committing to a core workout routine, Maria started to notice small changes. Her posture improved, she moved with greater ease, and, most importantly, she felt proud of herself for sticking with it. Maria's newfound strength boosted her confidence, making her feel more capable and self-reliant than she had in years.

The benefits of core workouts for seniors go far beyond just building physical strength. They improve balance and stability, enhance posture, reduce back pain, and boost confidence and independence. Whether it's helping you prevent falls, sit and stand with better posture, or simply feel more in control of your body, a strong core can transform your life.

As we've seen through stories like Helen, Tom, and Maria's, building core strength is not only achievable but can lead to profound improvements in your daily life. In the next chapter, we'll dive into specific core exercises designed for seniors, with variations to suit every fitness level. Together, we'll continue this journey toward ageless abs and a stronger, more confident you.

CHAPTER 4

AGELESS ABS: CORE WORKOUTS FOR SENIORS

Now that we've explored the benefits of a strong core and why it's essential as we age, it's time to dive into the heart of the matter: the exercises themselves. Building core strength doesn't have to be intimidating or out of reach, even for seniors who are new to working out or dealing with mobility challenges. In this chapter, you'll find a range of core exercises tailored to different fitness levels, from gentle beginner movements to advanced workouts for those ready to take on more. Whether you're starting small or looking to push yourself further, these exercises will help you build strength, stability, and confidence.

Beginner-Friendly Core Workouts

For those just starting on their core fitness journey, it's essential to ease into movements that build strength gradually without putting too much strain on the body. These beginner-friendly exercises are designed to target the muscles of the core while remaining gentle on joints and easy to follow.

Seated Marches

Seated marches are an excellent introduction to core engagement. Not only do they activate the abdominal muscles, but they also get the legs moving, helping with coordination and balance.

- How to do it: Sit up tall in a sturdy chair, feet flat on the floor and hands resting on your thighs. Slowly lift one knee toward your chest as if marching in place. Lower it back down and repeat with the other leg. Continue alternating for 10–15 reps on each leg.
- Tip: Focus on keeping your torso upright and your core engaged. Imagine drawing your belly button toward your spine with each march.

Pelvic Tilts

Pelvic tilts are another gentle exercise that strengthens the abdominal muscles while relieving tension in the lower back.

- How to do it: Lie on your back with your knees bent, feet flat on the floor. Place your hands on your hips. Slowly tilt your pelvis upward, flattening your lower back against the floor, then release back to the neutral position. Repeat for 10–12 reps.
- Tip: Keep the movement slow and controlled, focusing on tightening your abdominal muscles as you tilt your pelvis.

Lying Leg Raises

This classic core move is a great way to work your lower abdominals without putting stress on your back.

- How to do it: Lie on your back with your legs straight and arms by your sides. Slowly raise both legs toward the ceiling until they form a 90-degree angle with your torso. Lower them back down without letting your heels touch the floor. Repeat for 8–10 reps.

- Tip: If this feels too challenging, you can bend your knees slightly or raise one leg at a time.

Real-Life Success: Julia's Start

Julia, at 70, was new to core workouts and nervous about injuring herself. Starting with seated marches and pelvic tilts, she gradually built her strength. Within a few weeks, she noticed that getting up from chairs was easier, and she even felt more stable when walking.

Intermediate Core Workouts

Once you've built some foundational strength with the beginner exercises, you may be ready to take things up a notch. These intermediate workouts are more challenging, incorporating dynamic movements that engage multiple core muscles at once.

Bird-Dogs

The bird-dog exercise is fantastic for improving core strength and balance. It engages the muscles in your abdomen, lower back, and hips all at once.

- How to do it: Start on all fours, with your hands under your shoulders and knees under your hips. Extend your right arm forward and your left leg straight behind you, creating a straight line from hand to foot. Hold for a few seconds, then return to the starting position. Switch sides and repeat for 10 reps on each side.

- Tip: Keep your spine neutral and your gaze down, ensuring you're not arching your back during the movement.

Seated Knee Lifts

This exercise builds on the seated marches from the beginner level but adds a bit more challenge to target the core more intensely.

- How to do it: Sit tall in a chair with your hands gripping the sides for support. Lift both knees toward your chest simultaneously, engaging your lower abdominals. Hold for a moment, then lower your feet back to the floor. Repeat for 8–12 reps.
- Tip: Keep your core tight and avoid leaning back. If lifting both knees at once is too difficult, start with one leg at a time.

Plank Variations for Seniors

Planks are one of the most effective exercises for overall core strength, but they can be modified to suit seniors. A knee plank, for example, is a gentler version of the traditional plank.

- How to do it: Start on all fours with your forearms on the ground. Walk your feet back until your body forms a straight line from your shoulders to your knees. Hold this position for 10–20 seconds, gradually increasing your time as you get stronger.

- Tip: Focus on keeping your hips level and engaging your core throughout the exercise.

Real-Life Success: Bill's Progress

Bill, an active 65-year-old, had been doing beginner exercises for a while and was ready to step things up. Bird-dogs and plank variations became his go-to moves, and he found his posture improving and his lower back pain diminishing. He felt more agile and confident in his daily movements.

Advanced Core Workouts for the Active Senior

For seniors who are already fit and looking to push themselves further, advanced core exercises offer a great challenge. These moves require more strength and coordination but are highly effective in building a powerful core.

Side Planks

Side planks take the traditional plank to the next level by working the obliques, which are the muscles along the sides of your abdomen.

- How to do it: Lie on your side with your forearm on the floor, elbow directly under your shoulder. Stack your legs on top of each other, then lift your hips off the ground, forming a straight line from your head to your feet. Hold for 10–20 seconds, then switch sides.
- Tip: If holding this position feels too difficult, bend your knees and keep them on the floor for a modified version.

Stability Ball Crunches

For those comfortable using equipment, stability ball crunches can intensify core work by adding an element of instability, forcing your core muscles to work harder.

- How to do it: Sit on a stability ball with your feet flat on the floor. Walk your feet forward until your lower back is resting on the ball. Cross your arms over your chest and perform a crunch by lifting your upper body off the ball. Repeat for 8–10 reps.
- Tip: Keep your movements slow and controlled to maintain balance on the ball.

Dead Bugs

Dead bugs are a dynamic exercise that requires coordination and works both the upper and lower parts of the core.

- How to do it: Lie on your back with your arms extended toward the ceiling and your legs in a tabletop position (knees bent at 90 degrees). Lower your right arm and left leg toward the floor simultaneously, keeping your back flat on the ground. Return to the starting position and switch sides. Repeat for 10–12 reps.
- Tip: Move slowly and focus on keeping your lower back pressed into the floor to engage your core fully.

Real-Life Success: Anna's Advanced Challenge

Anna, a 67-year-old who had always been active, was looking for a way to keep her core workouts challenging. Incorporating side planks and stability ball crunches into her routine not only gave her a stronger core but also made her feel like she was defying the limitations that aging sometimes imposes.

Exercise Modifications for Common Mobility Issues

For seniors dealing with mobility issues, such as joint pain or arthritis, core workouts can still be highly effective with the right modifications. Here are some tips for adapting the exercises to suit different needs.

- Joint Pain: For those with sensitive knees or wrists, exercises like seated marches and knee planks provide a way to work the core without placing too much strain on joints.
- Limited Flexibility: If you find certain movements difficult due to limited flexibility, use props like a sturdy chair or cushions for support. For example, placing a cushion under your hips during pelvic tilts can make the exercise more comfortable.
- Arthritis: Stick to low-impact exercises, such as seated knee lifts and bird-dogs, which minimize stress on the joints while still effectively targeting the core.

Whether you're just starting or looking for a more advanced challenge, core workouts for seniors can be tailored to fit any fitness level or mobility need. The key is to start at your own pace and progress as you feel stronger. In the next chapter, we'll discuss how to create a personalized core workout plan that fits into your lifestyle, ensuring that you build lasting strength for years to come.

CHAPTER 5

BUILDING A BALANCED CORE ROUTINE

Creating a strong core is about more than just completing exercises—it's about developing a well-rounded approach that incorporates flexibility, strength, and endurance. A balanced core routine ensures that you don't just strengthen your abdominal muscles, but also improve your posture, protect your spine, and make daily activities easier. In this chapter, we'll guide you through the process of creating a weekly core workout plan that caters to your individual needs, while also teaching you how to track your progress in meaningful ways.

Combining Flexibility, Strength, and Endurance

Many people think of core workouts as solely strength-based, focusing on toning and building the muscles in the midsection. While strength is crucial, it's only one part of the equation. Flexibility and endurance play equally important roles, especially as we age.

Why Flexibility Matters

Flexibility in the core region ensures that muscles can move through their full range of motion without strain. Tightness in the hips or lower back can contribute to discomfort or even injury. Flexibility exercises, such as gentle stretches or yoga-inspired movements, help loosen tight muscles and improve overall mobility.

For example, simple stretches like the seated torso twist or the standing side bend can make a big difference in how limber you feel after your workouts. When combined with core-strengthening exercises, stretching can also prevent stiffness and promote a greater range of motion in your daily life.

Strength: The Foundation of Core Health

Core strength is the backbone (literally and figuratively) of any fitness routine, especially for seniors. By strengthening the muscles in your abdomen, lower back, and hips, you create a stable foundation that supports your spine, reduces the risk of injury, and helps you stay balanced during physical activities.

Endurance for Long-Term Benefits

Core endurance refers to your muscles' ability to work over time without becoming fatigued. You want your core muscles to not just be strong, but also able to support you through prolonged activities, whether it's a long walk, standing for an extended period, or playing with your grandkids. Building endurance ensures that your core muscles stay active and engaged throughout your daily routine, even when you're not consciously working them.

Real-Life Story: Joan's Balance of Strength and Flexibility

Joan, 72, started her core workout journey focusing on strength alone. After noticing some stiffness in her back and hips, she added flexibility exercises to her routine. Within a few weeks, she not only felt stronger but also more mobile, which made bending, twisting, and lifting much easier. The combination of strength, flexibility, and endurance has since allowed Joan to enjoy her active lifestyle without the stiffness she once experienced.

Creating a Weekly Core Workout Plan

No two people have the same fitness needs, so it's essential to develop a plan that's tailored to your level and goals. The good news is that it's easy to design a weekly workout routine that covers all the important aspects of core fitness—strength, flexibility, and endurance—without requiring hours of exercise each day.

Below, we outline sample weekly plans based on three fitness levels: beginner, intermediate, and advanced. Feel free to adjust them as needed based on how your body feels.

Beginner Core Workout Plan

- Day 1: Seated marches (2 sets of 15), pelvic tilts (2 sets of 10), lying leg raises (2 sets of 8)
- Day 2: Seated torso twist (2 sets of 10 per side), seated knee lifts (2 sets of 10), bird-dogs (2 sets of 8 per side)
- Day 3: Rest Day or light stretching (gentle back stretches, hip flexor stretch)
- Day 4: Seated marches (2 sets of 15), pelvic tilts (2 sets of 10), lying leg raises (2 sets of 8)
- Day 5: Gentle stretching or yoga (20–30 minutes)

- Day 6: Seated knee lifts (2 sets of 10), bird-dogs (2 sets of 8 per side), pelvic tilts (2 sets of 10)

- Day 7: Rest or go for a light walk (15–20 minutes)

Intermediate Core Workout Plan

- Day 1: Bird-dogs (3 sets of 10 per side), knee plank (2 sets, hold for 20 seconds), seated knee lifts (3 sets of 10)

- Day 2: Standing side bends (2 sets of 10 per side), lying leg raises (3 sets of 12), plank (2 sets, hold for 20 seconds)

- Day 3: Rest or light stretching

- Day 4: Bird-dogs (3 sets of 10 per side), knee plank (3 sets, hold for 30 seconds), lying leg raises (3 sets of 12)

- Day 5: Flexibility Day: yoga or Pilates-inspired stretching (30 minutes)

- Day 6: Plank (2 sets, hold for 20 seconds), seated knee lifts (3 sets of 10), standing side bends (2 sets of 10 per side)

- Day 7: Rest or light cardio (walking or swimming for 20–30 minutes)

Advanced Core Workout Plan

- Day 1: Side planks (3 sets, hold for 20–30 seconds per side), dead bugs (3 sets of 10 per side), bird-dogs (3 sets of 12)

- Day 2: Stability ball crunches (3 sets of 12), plank (3 sets, hold for 40 seconds), seated knee lifts (3 sets of 15)

- Day 3: Rest Day or flexibility work (30 minutes of deep stretches or yoga)

- Day 4: Side planks (3 sets, hold for 20–30 seconds per side), dead bugs (3 sets of 10 per side), plank (3 sets, hold for 40 seconds)

- Day 5: Flexibility Day with a focus on lower back and hip stretches (30–40 minutes)

- Day 6: Stability ball crunches (3 sets of 12), bird-dogs (3 sets of 12 per side), plank (3 sets, hold for 40 seconds)

- Day 7: Rest or a longer cardio session (walking, biking, or swimming for 30–40 minutes)

The key to success with any core workout plan is consistency. By working out regularly, you'll gradually build strength, flexibility, and endurance that will improve your overall quality of life. Remember that rest and recovery days are just as important as your workout days—they allow your muscles to rebuild and grow stronger.

Tracking Your Progress

Measuring your improvement over time helps you stay motivated and see the results of your hard work. For seniors, tracking progress doesn't always mean measuring your waistline or counting how many sit-ups you can do. Instead, focus on functional improvements and how you feel during your day-to-day life.

1. Improved Balance

One of the first signs of progress might be better balance. Have you noticed that you can walk longer distances without feeling unsteady? Or maybe you're able to reach for something on a high shelf without wobbling. These are subtle, but significant, indicators that your core is getting stronger.

2. Reduced Back Pain

A strong core takes the pressure off your lower back. If you experience chronic back pain, keep track of how often it occurs and how intense it is. Many seniors report a noticeable reduction in back pain after just a few weeks of consistent core exercises.

3. More Energy

Another way to gauge your progress is by how energetic you feel throughout the day. As your core strength improves, you may find yourself with more stamina to perform activities like walking, gardening, or even playing with your grandchildren.

4. Increased Independence

For many seniors, a major goal of core workouts is to maintain independence. Track how easily you're able to do things like getting up from a chair, climbing stairs, or carrying groceries. These activities become much easier as your core becomes stronger.

Real-Life Story: George's Milestones

George, 68, had always struggled with lower back pain and limited flexibility. After two months of following a consistent core workout plan, he noticed a significant decrease in his back pain. His balance improved so much that he could walk without his cane on most days, and his doctor remarked on how much more mobile he had become. George's success was a direct result of his commitment to tracking his progress and adjusting his routine as he grew stronger.

Building a balanced core routine that incorporates flexibility, strength, and endurance is the key to maintaining a healthy, functional body as you age. Whether you're just starting or already have an advanced fitness level, there's a plan that will work for you. The most important thing is to stay consistent and listen to your body. In the next chapter, we'll explore how to incorporate these core workouts into a broader fitness routine that promotes total-body wellness.

CHAPTER 6

STAYING MOTIVATED: OVERCOMING MENTAL AND PHYSICAL BARRIERS

Embarking on a fitness journey can feel overwhelming, especially for seniors who might be dealing with both physical limitations and mental hurdles. It's common to have doubts, concerns, and fears about starting a new exercise routine later in life. But just as the physical benefits of core workouts are clear, so too are the mental ones. Building a stronger core not only improves your physical health, but also boosts your confidence and mental well-being. In this chapter, we'll explore common mental barriers seniors face, and provide practical tips on how to stay motivated, build confidence, and seamlessly incorporate core exercises into daily life.

Common Mental Hurdles for Seniors Starting a Fitness Journey

Starting any new habit comes with challenges, and core workouts are no exception. For many seniors, the obstacles are as much mental as they are physical. It's natural to feel apprehensive, especially if you've been inactive for a while or have health concerns.

Fear of Injury

One of the biggest worries seniors faces when starting a fitness routine is the fear of getting hurt. With aging often comes more fragile bones and stiff joints, so it's understandable that the idea of physical exercise might feel risky. Many seniors shy away from core exercises because they assume they are too intense, or they may have had past experiences with pain or injury during exercise.

It's important to remember that core exercises, when done correctly, can actually reduce your risk of injury. Strengthening the muscles that support your spine, hips, and lower back improves stability and balance, which in turn helps prevent falls and other accidents. Start slow and focus on proper form to avoid strain, and always listen to your body—if something doesn't feel right, modify the exercise or take a break.

Lack of Energy

Feeling tired or sluggish is another common mental block that prevents many seniors from exercising. As we age, energy levels can dip, making the thought of exercising seem like an exhausting task. However, regular movement can actually increase your overall energy levels. It may seem counterintuitive, but physical activity stimulates the body's systems, helping you feel more alert and energized throughout the day.

Feeling Too Old to Start

It's easy to think, "I'm too old to start exercising now." This thought is particularly common for those who have been inactive for many years or who have health conditions that limit their movement. But the truth is, it's never too late to start focusing on your health. Countless seniors have found that starting a fitness routine in their 60s, 70s, or even 80s has transformed their mobility, reduced pain, and significantly improved their quality of life.

Real-Life Story: Barbara's Breakthrough

Barbara, a 74-year-old grandmother, had never been one for exercise. She often felt too tired and worried that working out might cause injury. But after her doctor recommended core strengthening exercises to help with her chronic lower back pain, she gave it a try. Starting slowly with seated marches and gentle stretches, Barbara found that not only did her back pain improve, but her energy levels increased as well. After a few weeks, she realized she could walk longer without feeling tired, and her fear of injury faded as she grew more confident in her abilities.

Building Confidence and Consistency

Staying committed to a new workout routine takes effort, especially when you're dealing with doubts or physical limitations. But building confidence in yourself and establishing consistency is key to long-term success.

Set Realistic Goals

One of the best ways to stay motivated is to set realistic, achievable goals. This doesn't mean aiming for six-pack abs or being able to run a marathon—it's about finding small, meaningful victories that keep you going. Perhaps your first goal is simply to complete a full week of core exercises. Once you reach that, you can set another goal, like holding a plank for 10 seconds longer than you did the week before.

By breaking down your larger fitness goals into smaller, manageable steps, you'll start to see progress faster, which will motivate you to keep going. Celebrate these wins, no matter how small they may seem. Each step forward is an achievement, and recognizing your progress builds both confidence and commitment.

Create a Routine You Enjoy

If exercise feels like a chore, it's going to be hard to stick with it. The key to staying consistent is finding a routine that you enjoy. Maybe you like the calm, focused nature of yoga-inspired core exercises, or perhaps you prefer a more active routine with standing movements that challenge your balance. Experiment with different exercises and routines until you find what works best for you.

Accountability and Support

Having someone to share your fitness journey with can also make a huge difference. Whether it's a workout buddy, a family member, or an online fitness community, having support helps you stay accountable and motivated. You don't have to do this alone—find someone who encourages you and shares in your successes.

Incorporating Core Workouts into Daily Life

Staying consistent doesn't mean you need to carve out a big chunk of your day for workouts. In fact, some of the best ways to strengthen your core are by incorporating exercises into your everyday activities. Here are a few practical tips for working core-strengthening movements into your daily routine.

Standing Tall

Good posture is one of the simplest and most effective ways to engage your core muscles throughout the day. Whenever you're standing—whether cooking, waiting in line, or chatting with friends—practice pulling your belly button toward your spine and standing tall with your shoulders back. This subtle movement engages your core and helps improve your posture over time.

Seated Core Exercises

If you spend a lot of time sitting, you can still activate your core muscles. Try seated knee lifts or seated marches while watching TV or reading. Even just sitting up straight with good posture engages your core and supports your spine.

Core Engagement During Daily Tasks

Think of your core as your body's foundation—it should be active during almost everything you do. When you bend down to pick something up, consciously engage your abdominal muscles to protect your back. If you're carrying groceries, focus on keeping your core tight as you walk. These small adjustments turn everyday movements into core-strengthening exercises.

Real-Life Story: John's Everyday Routine

John, 69, had always been active but found it hard to make time for dedicated workouts. Instead, he started incorporating core exercises into his daily routine. He practiced engaging his core while doing dishes, walking the dog, and even while driving. Over time, John noticed improvements in his posture and balance, and he felt stronger without needing to set aside time for long workouts.

Staying motivated is often the most challenging part of starting a fitness journey, but it's also the most rewarding. By addressing mental barriers, building confidence through small victories, and finding ways to incorporate core workouts into daily life, you can create a routine that is both sustainable and effective. Remember, every step you take is a step toward better health and independence. As you continue with your core workout routine, you'll not only build physical strength, but also mental resilience—setting yourself up for long-term success and improved well-being.

CHAPTER 7

LIFESTYLE FACTORS THAT SUPPORT CORE STRENGTH

Building a strong core goes beyond exercise; it's a holistic effort that includes attention to your overall lifestyle. From the food you eat to how you recover after workouts, the choices you make each day can significantly impact your strength and health. In this chapter, we'll explore three critical lifestyle factors—nutrition, hydration and recovery, and the mind-body connection—each of which plays a vital role in supporting your core workouts.

The Role of Nutrition in Muscle Health

A well-rounded diet is one of the most powerful tools in maintaining muscle health, especially as we age. As the body changes, the need for certain nutrients becomes more pronounced, and ensuring you are properly fueling your body can make a world of difference in how you feel, how you perform, and how well you maintain muscle strength—including your core muscles.

Protein: The Building Block of Muscle

One of the most important nutrients for maintaining and building muscle mass is protein. Protein provides the essential amino acids your muscles need to repair and grow stronger after exercise. For seniors, getting enough protein is particularly important, as muscle loss tends to accelerate with age—a condition known as sarcopenia.

A good rule of thumb is to include a source of protein with every meal. Lean meats like chicken or turkey, fish, eggs, dairy products, and plant-based proteins like beans, lentils, and tofu are all excellent choices. Even snacks can offer an opportunity to increase your protein intake—try adding nuts, seeds, or yogurt for a muscle-boosting snack.

Healthy Fats for Joint and Muscle Health

In addition to protein, healthy fats play an important role in keeping your body strong. Fats are essential for hormone regulation, which in turn impacts muscle growth and repair. Moreover, they support joint health by reducing inflammation, which is crucial for maintaining flexibility and preventing injury during exercise. Foods rich in omega-3 fatty acids, such as fatty fish (salmon, mackerel, sardines), walnuts, flaxseeds, and chia seeds, are particularly beneficial.

Vitamins and Minerals: The Unsung Heroes

Vitamins and minerals, often overlooked, are just as essential for muscle health. Calcium and vitamin D, for instance, are vital for bone strength and preventing osteoporosis—a concern for many seniors. Strong bones support a strong core, and ensuring you have enough calcium in your diet is key.

Magnesium is another important nutrient, as it helps with muscle function and energy production. You can find magnesium in leafy greens, nuts, and whole grains. Lastly, B-vitamins, found in foods like eggs, meat, and fortified cereals, are essential for energy metabolism, helping you stay energized throughout your workouts.

The Importance of Hydration and Recovery

While exercise and nutrition are often at the forefront of fitness discussions, hydration and recovery are equally important for achieving and maintaining core strength. Proper hydration and mindful recovery practices can make your core workouts more effective and help prevent injury.

Hydration: Fuel for Your Muscles

Water is essential for every bodily function, and staying hydrated is particularly important when you're working on building strength. Muscles are made up of about 75% water, and dehydration can lead to muscle cramps, fatigue, and reduced coordination—all of which can hamper your ability to perform core exercises effectively.

For seniors, staying hydrated can sometimes be challenging, especially if the body's thirst signals diminish with age. Aim to drink water regularly throughout the day, even if you don't feel particularly thirsty. A good indicator of proper hydration is the color of your urine—pale yellow usually means you're well-hydrated, while darker shades can indicate dehydration.

Incorporating hydrating foods, such as cucumbers, watermelon, and oranges, into your diet is another way to boost your fluid intake. And if you're exercising in warm weather or sweating a lot during workouts, consider adding a pinch of salt or an electrolyte supplement to your water to help with hydration balance.

Recovery: The Key to Building Strength

Recovery is where the magic happens. While workouts break down muscle fibers, recovery allows them to rebuild stronger. For seniors, proper recovery is crucial for preventing overuse injuries and muscle fatigue.

Stretching after your workout helps keep your muscles flexible and reduces soreness. Focus on stretching the major muscle groups that were worked during your core exercises, such as your abs, obliques, and lower back. You can also try gentle yoga or tai chi for a soothing post-workout routine that promotes relaxation and flexibility.

Rest days are just as important as workout days. Make sure to incorporate rest into your weekly routine—whether that means taking a full day off from exercise or engaging in light activities like walking or swimming. Rest doesn't mean inactivity, but rather allowing your body time to repair and rebuild itself, ensuring long-term progress and preventing burnout.

Mind-Body Connection: Yoga and Pilates for Core Strength

For many seniors, finding a fitness routine that strengthens both the body and the mind can be particularly rewarding. This is where practices like yoga and Pilates come into play. Both of these low-impact, senior-friendly options are excellent for building core strength, improving flexibility, and enhancing mental focus.

Yoga: Strength and Mindfulness

Yoga is a holistic practice that combines strength, flexibility, balance, and mindfulness, making it an ideal choice for seniors looking to build core strength while also enhancing their overall well-being. Many yoga poses focus on engaging the core muscles, even when you might not realize it. Poses such as Warrior II, Plank, and Boat Pose are all excellent for strengthening the abdominal muscles, lower back, and hips.

One of the benefits of yoga is that it can be easily modified to accommodate different fitness levels and mobility issues. Whether you're practicing on the mat or using a chair for support, yoga can be tailored to suit your needs. Beyond the physical benefits, yoga encourages mindfulness and stress reduction, both of which can enhance your overall mental and emotional health.

Pilates: Focused Core Training

While yoga emphasizes a balance between mind and body, Pilates is a system specifically designed to improve core strength. Developed by Joseph Pilates in the early 20th century, this method focuses on controlled movements that strengthen the body's "powerhouse" muscles—the abs, lower back, hips, and pelvic floor.

Many of the exercises in Pilates involve small, precise movements that deeply engage the core. For example, the Pelvic Curl, Leg Circles, and Hundreds are all classic Pilates exercises that target the core while also improving balance and coordination. Like yoga, Pilates can be modified to suit your fitness level and can be done on the floor or with the help of equipment like a Pilates reformer or a resistance band.

Real-Life Story: Eleanor's Transformation

Eleanor, 72, had always struggled with lower back pain and stiffness, which made traditional exercises difficult for her. After a friend recommended a gentle yoga class at her local community center, she decided to give it a try. At first, Eleanor was hesitant—she worried that she wouldn't be able to keep up with the class. But the instructor offered modifications for each pose, and Eleanor quickly found that she could comfortably participate. Over time, her core strength improved, and her back pain lessened significantly. She even began incorporating Pilates into her routine, giving her a newfound sense of strength and confidence in her daily life.

Building and maintaining core strength is about more than just exercise. It requires a lifestyle approach that includes proper nutrition, hydration, recovery, and a mindful connection between body and mind. By focusing on these essential lifestyle factors, you'll not only enhance your workouts but also improve your overall health and well-being. Through balanced nutrition, adequate hydration, thoughtful recovery, and practices like yoga and Pilates, you can support your body's journey toward ageless abs and a strong, resilient core.

CHAPTER 8

AVOIDING INJURY AND STAYING SAFE

As we age, staying safe during exercise becomes a top priority. While core workouts offer immense benefits, they also require mindfulness and care to avoid injury. For seniors, this is particularly important, as the risk of strain or overuse injuries may increase with age. In this chapter, we'll cover how to recognize the signs of overtraining, ensure correct form and posture, and understand when professional guidance might be necessary to keep your workouts safe and effective.

Recognizing the Signs of Overtraining

One of the most common mistakes people make—especially those eager to improve their fitness—is overtraining. It's easy to get swept up in the excitement of a new workout routine, but pushing your body too hard, too quickly, can lead to unnecessary injuries or setbacks.

Understanding Overtraining

Overtraining occurs when your body doesn't get enough rest between workouts to recover fully. For seniors, recovery time is especially important since muscles and joints take longer to heal than they did in younger years. The key is finding a balance between challenging your body and allowing it the time it needs to repair and grow stronger.

Warning Signs

The body has a way of signaling when it's had enough, and it's crucial to listen to those signals. Some common signs of overtraining include:

- Persistent muscle soreness that doesn't improve after a day or two

- Fatigue that lingers beyond your workout

- Decreased performance or feeling weaker during exercises that used to be easier

- Irritability or mood swings

- Trouble sleeping or feeling restless

- Aches in your joints, particularly in areas like the lower back, hips, or shoulders

Taking a Step Back

If you notice any of these signs, it's time to ease up. Remember, there's no rush when it comes to building core strength. Rest is an essential part of the process, allowing your muscles to repair and grow. Sometimes, taking a step back can actually accelerate your progress in the long run.

A good practice is to alternate between days of active exercise and days of lighter activity, such as walking or gentle stretching. This allows your body time to recover while keeping you moving.

Correct Form and Posture in Every Move

Proper form is the foundation of any exercise program, but it's especially important when it comes to core workouts. Poor form not only reduces the effectiveness of your exercises but also increases the risk of injury, particularly to the lower back and neck.

Engaging the Right Muscles

One of the most common mistakes in core exercises is relying on muscles other than your core to perform the movement. For instance, during exercises like crunches or leg lifts, many people unintentionally engage their hip flexors or strain their neck rather than activating their abdominal muscles. This can lead to discomfort or injury.

The key to correct form is making sure that the muscles you're targeting are the ones doing the work. In the case of core exercises, this means focusing on tightening your abdominal muscles, pulling your belly button in toward your spine, and maintaining a neutral spine position.

Basic Tips for Proper Posture

Here are a few general tips to ensure proper form during core exercises:

- Maintain a neutral spine: Whether you're lying on your back or standing, your spine should maintain its natural curve. This means avoiding overarching your lower back or rounding your shoulders forward.
- Avoid straining your neck: In exercises like crunches, keep your chin slightly tucked and your head aligned with your spine. Your hands should support, not pull, your head.

- Engage your core: Before you begin any core movement, consciously engage your abdominal muscles. Imagine you're trying to zip up a tight pair of pants—this helps activate your deep core muscles.

- Move slowly and with control: Rushing through exercises often leads to poor form. Instead, focus on slow, controlled movements. This not only reduces the risk of injury but also increases the effectiveness of the exercise by keeping your muscles engaged for longer.

Common Core Exercises and Correct Form

To help you get a better idea of what proper form looks like, here are some guidelines for common core exercises:

- Seated Marches: Sit tall in a chair with your feet flat on the floor. Engage your core and slowly lift one knee towards your chest, keeping your back straight. Lower your foot back down and repeat with the other leg.

- Pelvic Tilts: Lie on your back with your knees bent and feet flat on the floor. Gently tilt your pelvis upward, pressing your lower back into the floor while tightening your abdominal muscles. Hold for a few seconds, then relax.

- Planks: Start on your hands and knees, then extend your legs behind you so your body forms a straight line from head to heels. Keep your core tight and avoid letting your hips sag or rise too high. Hold for as long as you can with proper form.

Each of these exercises can be modified to suit your fitness level. For instance, if holding a plank is too challenging, you can perform it on your knees rather than your toes to reduce the strain on your core and lower back.

When to Seek Professional Guidance

Even with the best intentions, it can sometimes be hard to know if you're performing exercises correctly or if your body is responding well to your workouts. This is where professional guidance can be invaluable. Working with a fitness professional or physical therapist can help ensure you're exercising safely, especially if you have any pre-existing conditions or mobility issues.

Why Professional Help Can Make a Difference

Personal trainers and physical therapists are trained to assess your body's movement patterns and provide specific guidance on how to modify exercises to suit your needs. They can help you avoid common pitfalls, like overtraining or poor posture, and offer personalized advice based on your fitness level, goals, and any health concerns you might have.

For example, if you're dealing with arthritis, a professional can recommend exercises that strengthen your core without putting too much stress on your joints. If you've recently had surgery or are recovering from an injury, they can provide modifications and exercises that support your healing process while still working on core strength.

Knowing When to Ask for Help

Here are a few scenarios in which seeking professional guidance may be a good idea:

- You're new to exercise: If you're just starting your fitness journey, a professional can help you develop a safe and effective workout plan tailored to your needs.

- You have a pre-existing condition: If you have arthritis, osteoporosis, back issues, or any other health concerns, a physical therapist can help you navigate exercises safely.

- You're recovering from injury: If you've experienced a fall, surgery, or any injury, working with a therapist can ensure that your exercise routine supports recovery without causing further damage.

- You're unsure about your form: If you've been exercising but aren't sure if you're doing it correctly, a trainer can provide valuable feedback on your form and technique.

Real-Life Story: John's Journey to Injury-Free Workouts

John, 68, had always been active, but after an injury to his lower back, he found it difficult to get back into a workout routine. Every time he tried, his back pain would flare up, making him hesitant to continue. Frustrated, he sought the help of a physical therapist, who worked with him to develop a modified core workout plan. With professional guidance, John was able to strengthen his core muscles without aggravating his back, and he's now able to enjoy his daily activities without pain.

Staying safe during core workouts is all about listening to your body and respecting its limits. By recognizing the signs of overtraining, maintaining proper form, and seeking professional help when needed, you can enjoy the benefits of core exercises without the risk of injury. Whether you're just starting or looking to improve your current routine, safety should always be your top priority. Remember, the goal is progress, not perfection, and with mindful practice, you can build a strong, resilient core that supports your overall health and well-being.

CHAPTER 9

SUCCESS STORIES: REAL-LIFE EXAMPLES OF SENIORS ACHIEVING AGELESS ABS

As with any fitness journey, the path to stronger core muscles and a healthier body is filled with both challenges and rewards. In this chapter, we'll take a look at real-life examples of seniors who have embraced core workouts and transformed their lives. These stories demonstrate that it's never too late to improve your strength, stability, and overall well-being, no matter your age. Through dedication, persistence, and some smart adjustments, these seniors have defied expectations and achieved remarkable results. Let their stories inspire you to continue your own journey toward "Ageless Abs."

Inspiring Transformations

Martha's Story: A Return to Independence

Martha, 72, had always prided herself on being active and independent. But after a bad fall in her late 60s, she struggled with balance and mobility, leaving her reliant on others for simple tasks like grocery shopping or going for a walk in her neighborhood. Determined to regain her freedom, Martha began working on her core strength.

At first, she found the exercises challenging—her muscles were weak, and her body daily resisted movement in ways it hadn't before. But with the help of a physical therapist and a routine of seated marches, pelvic tilts, core exercises, Martha's strength gradually returned.

Within a few months, her balance had significantly improved, and she noticed she could stand taller and move with more confidence.

By the time she turned 73, Martha no longer feared falling, and she was back to running errands on her own. "I feel like I've been given a second chance," she says. "My core has brought me back to the life I love."

Henry's Journey: From Stiffness to Strength

Henry, 65, spent much of his life behind a desk. After retiring, he noticed that his posture was poor, and his back often ached after simple activities like bending over to tie his shoes. He had always assumed that such stiffness and discomfort were just part of getting older. But a chance conversation with his doctor made him realize that his core muscles were weak and that strengthening them could help alleviate his back pain.

Henry started small, doing beginner core exercises like lying leg lifts and pelvic tilts. Over time, as his core became stronger, he added in bird-dogs and seated knee lifts to challenge himself further. It wasn't an easy journey—there were days when his muscles felt sore, and he doubted whether the effort was worth it. But slowly, he noticed the pain in his lower back fading.

Now, Henry stands taller, walks with more ease, and is even considering taking up golf. "I never thought I'd see the day when I could move without pain," Henry says. "Strengthening my core has changed everything."

Challenges and Triumphs

Gloria's Path: Overcoming Arthritis

At 78, Gloria had lived with arthritis for more than a decade. The pain in her joints, especially in her hips and knees, made it difficult for her to stay active, and she feared that any attempt at exercise would only make her arthritis worse. But after attending a workshop on fitness for seniors, Gloria decided to try a gentle core workout program designed specifically for people with arthritis.

The beginning was tough—Gloria struggled with stiffness, and her joints would ache after her sessions. But with the guidance of her instructor, she learned how to modify the exercises to suit her body's needs. She incorporated light resistance bands and stability balls to reduce the strain on her joints while still working on her core muscles.

After a few months, Gloria started noticing real changes. Her movements became smoother, and she found that she could go about her daily routine with less pain. "It wasn't easy," she admits, "but sticking with it has made such a difference. I feel like I've taken control of my arthritis rather than letting it control me."

Paul's Triumph: Reclaiming His Confidence

Paul, 69, had always been a strong and active man, working in construction for most of his life. But after retiring, his activity levels dropped, and over time, he began to gain weight and lose strength. His once-powerful body now felt sluggish and weak, and he started to lose confidence in his ability to do the things he once enjoyed, like playing with his grandchildren or taking long walks with his wife.

Feeling frustrated, Paul decided to make a change. He signed up for a senior fitness class at his local community center, where he was introduced to core workouts. At first, he found them surprisingly difficult—his balance was off, and his abs seemed to have forgotten how to engage. But Paul wasn't one to give up easily.

With consistent effort, Paul gradually regained his strength. He started with beginner exercises but quickly progressed to more advanced moves like side planks and dead bugs. The improvements weren't just physical—Paul's confidence soared as he realized he was capable of more than he had thought possible. "It's not just about the muscles," Paul says. "It's about feeling good in my own skin again."

Now, Paul is back to chasing after his grandchildren and walking with his wife every morning. His core workouts have helped him reclaim his sense of vitality, and he's never felt better.

Testimonials of Commitment

Margaret's Testimony: The Power of Consistency

Margaret, 74, had always been active in her younger years, but as time passed, she found it harder to keep up with regular exercise. When her doctor recommended core workouts to improve her balance and prevent falls, Margaret was skeptical. She wasn't sure she had the energy or discipline to stick with a new routine. However, she decided to give it a try, starting with just 10 minutes of core exercises a day.

At first, progress felt slow, and there were days when she didn't feel like doing the exercises at all. But Margaret stuck with it, reminding herself that consistency was key. Week by week, she noticed small improvements—her balance was better, and she didn't tire as easily when doing household chores.

After a few months, Margaret's efforts paid off in a big way. Not only was she stronger, but she felt more energized and capable in her daily life. "It's not about doing a lot at once," Margaret says. "It's about showing up every day, even when it's hard."

Frank's Testimony: Core Workouts as a Lifeline

Frank, 70, was diagnosed with Parkinson's disease five years ago, and as his condition progressed, he found it increasingly difficult to maintain his strength and coordination. His doctor suggested core workouts to help him stay mobile and manage his symptoms, but Frank was hesitant. He feared that his condition would make it impossible to exercise without hurting himself.

With the help of a physical therapist, Frank began a carefully tailored core workout program that included exercises designed to improve his balance and stability. The journey wasn't easy, but Frank persisted, determined to hold onto his independence for as long as possible.

Today, Frank credits his core workouts with helping him maintain a sense of control over his body. "Parkinson's is part of my life, but it doesn't define me," Frank says. "Working on my core has given me strength—not just physically, but mentally too."

These stories of transformation show that it's never too late to start building a stronger core and improving your quality of life. The challenges are real, but so are the rewards. Whether you're overcoming injury, arthritis, or just the everyday effects of aging, core workouts can help you regain control of your body, boost your confidence, and feel more empowered in your daily life. The key is to stay consistent, listen to your body, and celebrate every step of progress along the way. If these seniors can do it, so can you.

CHAPTER 10

SUSTAINING CORE STRENGTH FOR THE LONG TERM

Building core strength is one thing—maintaining it over the long term is quite another. As with any fitness journey, consistency is the key to reaping lasting benefits. After dedicating time and effort to strengthening your core, it's important to think about how you can maintain those gains for years to come. Whether you're managing new physical challenges or simply looking for ways to stay motivated, this chapter will help you sustain the progress you've made and continue your journey toward lifelong fitness.

Maintaining Your Gains: Staying Strong and Active as You Age

As we grow older, the body inevitably changes. Muscles naturally lose mass, joints become stiffer, and energy levels fluctuate more than they once did. However, this doesn't mean that you can't stay strong and active well into your senior years. The good news is that by maintaining a regular core workout routine, you can hold onto your strength and mobility while minimizing age-related decline.

The key to preserving core strength lies in consistency. Just like brushing your teeth or taking your daily vitamins, think of core exercises as a non-negotiable part of your routine. You don't have to spend hours working out each day—a few minutes of targeted movements, combined with an active lifestyle, will help maintain the strength you've built. Incorporating exercises that focus on all aspects of the core—abs, obliques, lower back, and hips—will ensure that your entire midsection stays strong, balanced, and capable.

New physical challenges may arise, such as arthritis flare-ups, joint pain, or decreased flexibility. But instead of seeing these obstacles as reasons to stop, view them as opportunities to adjust and adapt. For instance, if your hips feel stiff, try gentle stretches to loosen them up before diving into more intense movements. If balance becomes a concern, focus on stability exercises that keep you grounded, like seated marches or slow, controlled side leg raises. Remember, the goal is to work with your body, not against it.

Keeping Core Workouts Fun and Engaging

One of the best ways to ensure you stick with your core workout routine is to keep things fun and engaging. Just because core exercises are important doesn't mean they have to be boring! Variety is essential to preventing burnout and keeping your workouts enjoyable. Here are a few ways to spice up your routine:

- Switch Up Your Exercises: It's easy to get stuck doing the same movements over and over, but incorporating new exercises can keep you motivated and challenge your muscles in different ways. If you've mastered seated knee lifts and pelvic tilts, try adding in new movements like plank variations or side leg raises. If you're already doing intermediate exercises like bird-dogs, consider moving on to more advanced exercises like side planks or dead bugs. Keeping your muscles guessing will help you avoid plateaus and keep the progress coming.

- Partner Up: Working out with a buddy can make exercise more social and enjoyable. Whether it's a friend, spouse, or fellow senior at your local community center, having someone to share your fitness journey with can provide motivation and accountability. On days when you're feeling low on energy or just not in the mood to exercise, knowing that someone else is counting on you to show up can be a powerful incentive.

- Join a Class: If you're someone who thrives in a group setting, consider joining a senior fitness class that includes core work. Many community centers, gyms, and online platforms offer group workouts specifically designed for older adults. Not only will you benefit from the expertise of an instructor, but you'll also have the camaraderie of exercising with others who are on a similar journey.

- Mix in Some Fun Activities: Remember that core strength can also be built outside of a traditional workout setting. Dancing, swimming, tai chi, and even gardening all engage your core muscles in different ways. By participating in activities you enjoy, you'll continue to build strength while having fun—and you may not even realize you're working out!

Setting New Goals for Lifelong Fitness

Fitness is a lifelong journey, and setting goals can help you stay motivated, focused, and excited about what's to come. While your initial goal may have been to build a stronger core, once you've reached that point, it's important to keep setting new targets to continue growing and improving.

Consider what aspects of your fitness you'd like to work on next. Perhaps you'd like to improve your flexibility or posture. Maybe you're interested in trying new forms of exercise, like Pilates or yoga, which can complement your core work. Or perhaps you'd like to challenge yourself by increasing the intensity or duration of your core workouts.

Setting specific, measurable, and attainable goals is key. For example, you might set a goal to hold a plank for 30 seconds or to complete three sets of side planks twice a week. As you achieve these milestones, celebrate your progress and use it as fuel to keep pushing forward.

It's also important to recognize that fitness goals can shift over time, especially as your body changes with age. Your goals in your 70s or 80s might look different from those you had in your 50s or 60s, and that's perfectly okay. Fitness is not about perfection; it's about progress. As long as you're moving, challenging yourself, and staying committed to your health, you're on the right track.

Sustaining core strength is not just about maintaining muscle tone or achieving a certain level of fitness; it's about living a life filled with vitality, independence, and confidence. By staying committed to your core workout routine, keeping things fun and varied, and setting new goals along the way, you can continue to enjoy the many benefits of a strong core well into your golden years.

Remember, this journey is yours to shape. Whether you're tackling new physical challenges, finding joy in group workouts, or celebrating small victories, every step you take brings you closer to a life of strength, stability, and well-being. Core strength isn't just for the young—it's for anyone who wants to live with strength and grace at any age. You've already come so far—now keep going!

CONCLUSION

As you've worked through this book, you've taken an important step toward improving your strength, stability, and overall well-being. The journey to building and maintaining core strength is about much more than achieving flat stomach or toned abs—it's about empowering yourself to live with confidence, grace, and independence at every age.

already

Whether you're just starting your fitness journey or have made great strides, the most important thing to remember is that progress comes in many forms. It could be the newfound ease with which you rise from a chair, the improvement in your posture, or the increased energy you feel throughout the day. These victories, large and small, are proof of your dedication and determination.

Aging brings its own set of challenges, but it also brings wisdom and resilience. You've learned how to listen to your body, how to push past mental and physical barriers, and how to adapt exercises to meet your needs. Core strength is a lifelong investment in your health, and you have laid a strong foundation for the years to come. Embrace the process, take pride in your progress, and continue to nurture your strength.

The key to sustaining this journey is consistency, but also joy. Find joy in movement, celebrate the small wins, and remember that it's never too late to set new goals. Whether you're continuing to improve your core strength or exploring new areas of fitness, your journey is ongoing—and it's one you should feel proud of.